MW01293288

This Book Belongs To:

Made in the USA
Las Vegas, NV
19 July 2024

92590546R00066